Trauma & Casualty Care for Law Enforcement and First Responders (TCC-LEFR)

Editors:

Wilfred Chapleau, R.N., EMT-P

Greg Chapman, B.S., R.R.T., REMT-P

Michael J. Hunter, EMT-P, TP-C

Peter T. Pons, M.D., F.A.C.E.P.

Lance Stuke, M.D., F.A.C.S.

International PreHospital Medicine Institute

Paperback ISBN: 978-1-7344044-4-9
Ebook ISBN: 978-1-7344044-2-5

IPHMI MISSION STATEMENT

The mission of the International PreHospital Medicine Institute is to provide relevant, timely, up to date, and affordable information and education to providers of prehospital medicine worldwide.

ACKNOWLEDGEMENTS

The information in TCC-LEFR was adapted from the United States Military Tactical Combat Casualty Care Course by the E.M.S. Education Department of the Denver Health Paramedic Division in cooperation with Denver Police Metro S.W.A.T. Unit and is consistent with the guidelines of Tactical Emergency Casualty Care.

This educational program would not have been possible without the efforts of James Manson, EMT-P, former EMS Education Chief at the Denver Paramedic Division, Denver Health and Hospital Authority whose vision and support allowed for the pilot TCC-LEFR program, Jesse Jerome, EMT-P and Jeff McMullen, EMT-P who assisted with curriculum development and course presentation, and James Robinson, EMT-P, former Assistant EMS Chief, whose advocacy allowed for the dissemination of this information throughout the Denver Metropolitan area and its public safety agencies as well as elsewhere in the US and the world.

The Editors would like to acknowledge the contributions of Ms. Tamara Cribley from The Deliberate Page for her invaluable assistance and tireless effort formatting this material and preparing it for publication. Thank you for all of the hard work you put in to make this a publication reality.

This book is dedicated to all public safety responders in law enforcement, the fire service, and emergency medical services who selflessly serve the public often at great personal sacrifice.

DISCLAIMER

The practice of emergency care in the out-of-hospital setting is ever-changing and evolving. As practice experience and research expand our knowledge base, changes in prehospital practice and the care provided may be necessary.

It is the responsibility of every individual providing prehospital care to determine the most appropriate management for any given patient in accordance with their training, scope of practice, and local procedures and protocols.

To the extent allowed by law, the publisher and authors do not assume any liability for any injury or damage to any patient or person as a result of information obtained from this educational program.

Remember that you must practice within your authorized scope of practice. Only do what you are authorized to do within your agency and community

ABOUT THE EDITORS

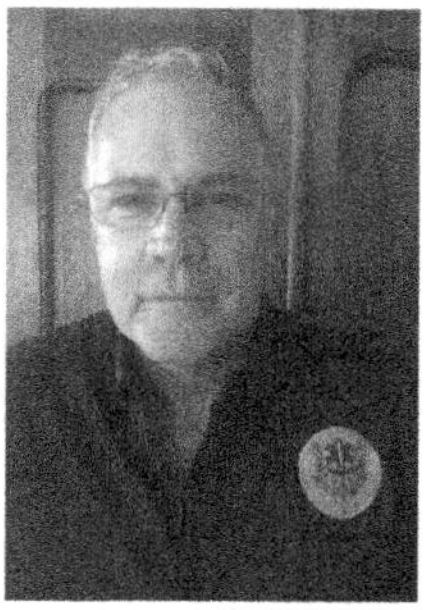

Will Chapleau has been a Paramedic for 41 years and trauma nurse specialist for 28 years. For the last five years he has served as the Director of Performance Improvement at the American College of Surgeons after spending 6 years managing Trauma training programs for the Committee on Trauma there. He also spent 20 years with the Chicago Heights Fire Department, the last 6 years as Chief. He also spent 15 years as an educator in the Good Samaritan Hospital EMS System in Downers Grove, Ill., and at St. James Hospital and Prairie State College in Chicago Heights. Chapleau served as the Chair of the PHTLS Committee of NAEMT for nearly 20 years. He also served on the NAEMT Board of Directors, as well as on the boards for the National Association of EMS Educators and the Society of Trauma Nurses. He also chaired a task force for the National Association of EMS Physicians. He's been a frequent contributor to the Journal of Emergency Medical Services (JEMS), EMS World Magazine and Fire Apparatus Magazine. He has also been published in the Journal of Trauma and Critical Care and the Journal of Emergency Medicine. He also served on the editorial board of EMS World Magazine. Will has written and edited five pre-hospital care texts in four languages and has taught prehospital care and lectured in conferences in over 60 countries.

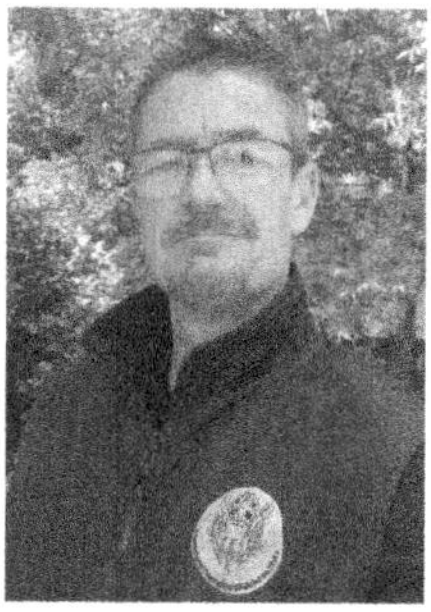

Greg Chapman a paramedic, Respiratory Therapist and Educator has been involved in EMS since 1975, holds a baccalaureate degree from the State University of New York in Economics and Educational Administration. He has worked in all aspect of public safety from EMS, Law Enforcement and Fire Service and brings a multifaceted view to the table. He served as a member of the Prehospital Trauma Life Support (PHTLS) Committee for over 20 years. He was responsible for the development of multiple editions of trauma and tactical courses. Chapman serves on the Board of Advisors of the Committee for Tactical Emergency Casualty Care, charged with the development of Standards used in the austere environments that we now face. Chapman has 30 years as a professional Ski Patroller and served on many SAR teams. Chapman has given presentations and seminars worldwide in over 20 countries and is published in multiple journals and textbooks. Chapman serves as a site visitor for the CoAEMSP and strongly believes that exceptional primary education is the cornerstone for the growth of EMS as a profession.

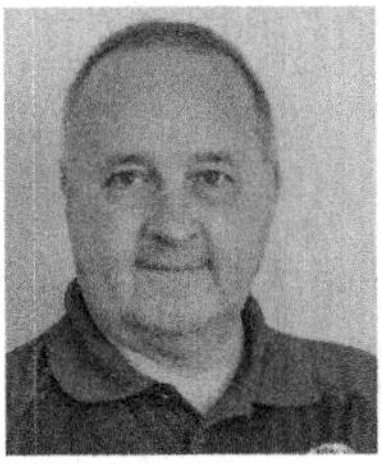

Michael J. Hunter, a veteran of EMS for more than 37 years, serves as Deputy Chief EMS for Worcester EMS (WEMS) at UMass Memorial Medical Center (UMMMC) University Campus in Worcester, Mass., where he has worked for more than 25 years. Hunter also functions as a tactical paramedic (TP-C #77) for WEMS and is assigned to the Massachusetts State Police STOP Team medical support group. He has served on the Massachusetts Committee of Trauma's Trauma Registry Sub-Committee and is an active member of the UMMHC Emergency Medicine/Trauma Committee. He is active in regional disaster planning, sits on the Central Mass EMS Corporation's Board of Directors and a is member of the Regional Medical Services Committee. Hunter was a founding member of the WEMS Honor Guard. Hunter is a long-standing member of NAEMT and served as a past member of their PHTLS Committee. He is also a charter member of the International Association of EMS Chiefs, a professional member of the National Association of EMS Physicians and the Special Operations Medical Association.

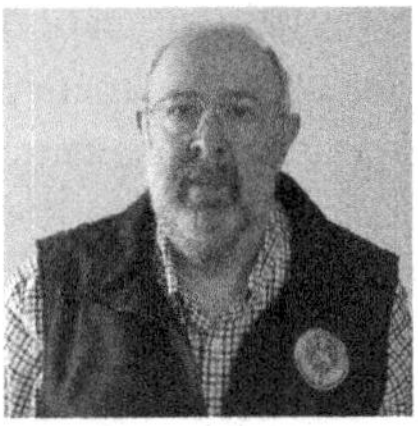

Peter T. Pons, M.D. is a board certified emergency physician in Denver, Colorado and has been actively involved with prehospital care and disaster preparedness for over 40 years. He was the E.M.S. Medical Director for the 9-1-1 paramedic ambulance service in Denver based at Denver Health. In addition, he has served as the E.M.S. physician director for the fire-based EMS systems of Glendale, Colorado and Jacksonville, Florida. He serves as an educator and the physician director of the tactical casualty care educational programs (Tactical Combat Casualty Care, Tactical Emergency Casualty Care, and Tactical Casualty Care for Law Enforcement and First Responders) offered by the EMS Education department of the Denver Paramedics. He has published numerous peer-reviewed journal articles on EMS, contributed many chapters for textbooks related to emergency medicine, and edited several textbooks for EMTs and Paramedics. He has served as the physician director for numerous mass gatherings and special events in Denver including the Denver Grand Prix, World Youth Day and the Visit of Pope John Paul II. He has lectured nationally and internationally on EMS, served as a member and chair of the EMS Committee for the American College of Emergency Physicians, and was a member of the Board of Directors for the American Board of Emergency Medicine.

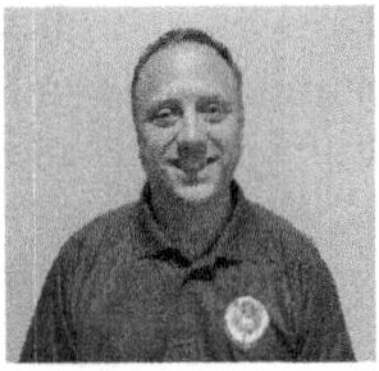

Lance Stuke, M.D. is a trauma surgeon at the Norman E. McSwain, Jr Spirit of Charity Trauma Center at University Medical Center, is an Associate Professor of Surgery at LSU, and serves as the Program Director for the LSU General Surgery residency. Prior to attending medical school he worked for several years as a paramedic for the City of New

Orleans. He attended medical school at Tulane University, completed a general surgery residency at the University of Texas-Southwestern/Parkland Hospital in Dallas, and returned to New Orleans for his trauma/critical care fellowship at LSU. He is a member of the EMS Committee of the American College of Surgeons Committee on Trauma and serves on the State of Louisiana EMS Certifying Commission. He has a research interest in prehospital trauma, has written numerous textbook chapters on prehospital trauma care, and lectured at many national and international prehospital conferences.

TABLE OF CONTENTS

TRAUMA AND CASUALTY CARE FOR LAW ENFORCEMENT AND FIRST RESPONDERS

1. INTRODUCTION:

The focus of this educational material is on the recognition of life threatening injuries with appropriate medical treatment in a tactical or other hazardous environment. This training will show you the actions that you can take to save a life – yours, your partner's, or any other injured individual – before EMS can get to or enter a dangerous scene.

While this material focuses primarily on tactical situations and any resulting injury, the medical care principles discussed apply to any and all trauma situations such a motor vehicle crashes, falls, assaults, work-related incidents, etc.

Military Information in this Course:

Much of the information in this course comes directly from medical research done by the Unites States military on the battlefields of Iraq and Afghanistan. While there are obvious differences between the battlefield setting and the civilian tactical setting, the basic operational medicine is the same. The specific situation will dictate how the principles of care are applied.

Why do I need to learn about this?

Because after someone sustains a traumatic injury, whether at home, at work, as a result of an accident, or as the result of intentional injury, the single most common cause of death that could have been prevented is…***UNCONTROLLED BLEEDING***

Causes of Preventable Death after Trauma in the Military

Viet Nam:

- The number 1 cause of preventable death was bleeding from arm or leg wounds
- The number 2 cause was from tension pneumothorax which interferes with breathing and circulation
- The number 3 cause was from an obstruction of the airway

The most important point is that ALL of these problems could have been treated effectively in the field.

Iraq and Afghanistan:

- In one study of 232 patients, uncontrolled bleeding was the cause of death in 85%
- Of those cases, one-third could have been treated in the field

Importance of the First Responder

In the military, 75-90% of all combat deaths occur before the casualty ever reaches a Medical Treatment Facility (MTF). The following statement was made over 120 years ago in 1898 by Col. Nicholas Senn, M.D. and is still true today:

> *"The fate of the wounded lies in the hands of the ones who apply the first dressing"*

The first person who reaches an injured patient and who can stop the bleeding is going to save a life. In the military, that is the corpsman, medic, pararescueman (PJ), Combat Lifesaver or all non-medical combatants. In the civilian setting that should include every public safety responder, including EMS, firefighters, and police officers. Ideally, every citizen would be trained in these principles so that they too can initiate care.

By teaching these trauma care principles in the military, the result is the best casualty treatment and survival in history. In fact, the death rate for wounded soldiers has been cut in half from World War II to Viet Nam and now, Iraq and Afghanistan. These same medical care principles taught in the military also apply to the civilian setting and will help to keep an injured patient alive long enough to get to a trauma center to receive the definitive care they require.

The Three Primary Objectives of TCC-LEFR

- Complete the mission – regardless of the type of threat, completing the mission means dealing with the threat or hazard
- Treat any and all casualties
- Prevent additional casualties

The goal of tactical situation management can be represented by the acronym "*T.H.R.E.A.T.*"

T. stands for **Threat suppression.** Anytime there is a threat, whether it is from something like an active shooter situation or any other kind of danger, the threat must be contained or controlled in order to provide medical care in relative safety.

H. stands for **Hemorrhage control**. As already mentioned, the most common cause of preventable death after injury is uncontrolled bleeding. Therefore the number one priority is to control any and all life-threatening external bleeding in a trauma victim.

R.E. stands for **Rapid Extrication** to safety. As soon as it is practical given the potential threat, a trauma victim should be extricated to a location of relative safety where medical care can be provided.

A. stands for **Assessment** by medical providers. The ideal situation is to have extricated the injured individual to a location where medical providers from the Emergency Medical Services (EMS) system can evaluate the patient's injuries and provide necessary life-saving interventions.

T. stands for **Transport** to definitive care. There are some injuries, particularly those that are located inside the chest or abdomen, which cannot be managed in the field. In those cases, it is important to expeditiously transport the patient to a facility that can treat those injuries. Typically, this means transporting the injured patient to a trauma center where all of the resources necessary to control internal bleeding.

Ideally, the management of a tactical or hazardous situation with injured individuals would proceed as follows:

1. Stabilize the tactical situation so EMS responders can enter the scene and treat the patient.

   - *If that is not possible:*

2. Evacuate the patient to a location where the individual can safely receive care by the EMS responders

   - *If that is not possible:*

3. Provide treatment for life-threatening medical problems within your training and scope of practice as the hazardous situation allows

   A. Stop the bleeding

   - Apply a Tourniquet
   - Pack the wound and apply direct pressure

   B. Open an obstructed airway

   C. Recognize increasing trouble breathing (tension pneumothorax)

2. WOUNDING PATTERNS & HEMORRHAGE

Injuries and wounds to the body can be characterized based upon their location.

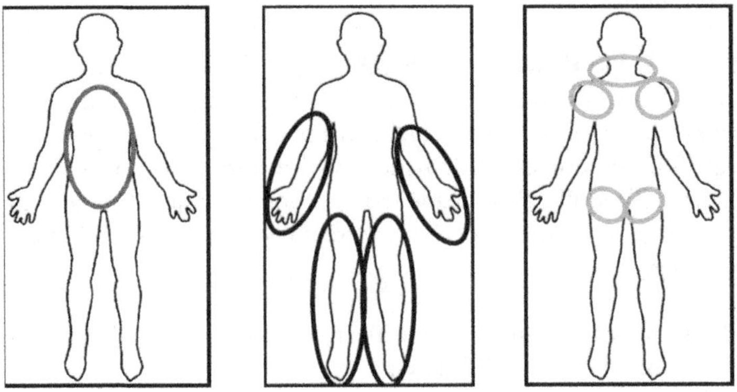

Central Wounds

- Central wounds are those that involve the central part of the body (the trunk). This includes the chest, back, abdomen, and pelvis.
- In all of these cases, most of the bleeding is occurring internally within the chest, abdominal and pelvic cavities.
- This internal bleeding *CANNOT* be controlled in field. The only place this bleeding will be managed is in the operating room of a trauma center.
- Therefore, these patients need rapid extrication from the site of injury for emergency transport to the trauma center.
- Identify these patients to the arriving paramedics so they can expedite their evaluation and transport.

There are several wound locations that can be the cause of preventable death but which *CAN* be treated in the field:

Limb Wounds

Wounds of the limbs (arms and legs) should have any bleeding controlled in the field.

Junctional Wounds

Wounds located in junctional areas, which are the sites where the head, arms, and legs join with the central part of the body (trunk) have a number of things in common:

- They all have a large artery that is located near the surface
    - Neck – carotid artery
    - Shoulder and armpit – axillary artery
    - Groin – femoral artery
- All have a boney structure located beneath against which a bleeding artery can be compressed in order to control the bleeding

Additional injuries that can be recognized and managed in the field include:

- Tension pneumothorax, and
- Airway obstruction

These will be discussed in more detail in later sections.

3. PHASES OF CARE IN TCC-LEFR: TIMING IS EVERYTHING

Casualty scenarios in a hazardous situation pose two major problems:

- A medical problem, and
- A tactical problem

The goal is try to assure the best possible outcome for both the casualty and the mission

Good medicine can sometimes be bad tactics. Bad tactics can get more people injured or killed or cause the mission to fail

Doing the **RIGHT THING** at the **RIGHT TIME** is critical

TCC-LEFR divides providing medical care into 3 phases based on the tactical situation or hazard. When there is an immediate hazard, attention is focused primarily on dealing with or eliminating the threat. As the threat or hazard decreases, additional medical care can be provided to a casualty. The three phases of care have been described using both military terminology and non-military terminology.

The military terminology is based upon the Tactical Combat Casualty Care Course and guidelines.

- Care Under Fire
- Tactical Field Care
- Tactical Evacuation Care

The non-military terminology is based upon the civilian all-hazards Tactical Emergency Casualty Care guidelines.

Direct Threat Care

- Indirect Threat care
- Evacuation Care

Care Under Fire (CUF) or Direct Threat Care

- This refers to the medical care rendered by the first responder at the scene of the injury while still under an immediate threat.
- Available medical equipment is limited to that carried by the individual or by the medical provider in his or her aid bag.
- Typically, this phase of care is primarily either self-care or buddy care if working as a team.

Tactical Field Care (TFC) or Indirect Threat Care

- This phase of care refers to the medical care provided by the first responder once there is no longer an immediate threat and the hazard has been controlled or contained.
- This phase of care also applies to situations in which an injury has occurred, but there is no imminent danger.
- Available medical equipment is still limited to that carried into the field by unit personnel
- Time to extrication and evacuation to a medical treatment facility may vary considerably depending upon location and incident circumstances.

Tactical Evacuation Care (TEC) or Evacuation Care

- This phase of care refers to the care rendered once the casualty has been picked up for evacuation and transport.
- Additional medical personnel and equipment are available in this phase of casualty management.
- This phase of care is similar to standard emergency medical care.

For purposes of this educational material and Trauma and Casualty Care for Law Enforcement and First Responders, the military terminology will be primarily used, although both the TCCC and TECC terms may appear.

4. M.A.R.C.H.

The U.S. Military developed an acronym (M.A.R.C.H.) designed to serve as an easy way to remember the most important steps to take medically when dealing with an injured individual. The M.A.R.C.H. acronym defines the general approach to and priorities for care of a trauma patient.

- **M**assive hemorrhage

  Life-threatening bleeding should be controlled as soon as possible.

- **A**irway

  An open airway should be established and maintained.

- **R**espiration (Breathing)

  - Open chest wounds that are bubbling or sucking air should be sealed
  - A possible tension pneumothorax, which is a life-threatening problem, should be recognized and the suspicion reported immediately to arriving EMS responders.

- **C**irculation

  All other bleeding should be controlled.

- **H**ypothermia/**H**ead injury

  - Prevent/treat hypothermia (decreased body temperature)
  - Recognize the signs of a possible head injury.

5. CARE UNDER FIRE - DIRECT THREAT CARE

Care Under Fire Guidelines

- Control the threat or hazard
  - If the situation involves an active shooter, law enforcement should return fire and all should take cover

- If a casualty is sustained but the wound is minor, the casualty may remain involved in the response to the incident if able and appropriate
- If a casualty is sustained and the wound is significant, direct the casualty to move to cover and apply self-aid if able
- Try to keep the casualty from sustaining additional wounds
- Stop *life-threatening* external hemorrhage if tactically feasible:
  - Direct the casualty to control hemorrhage by self-aid if able
  - Apply an approved tourniquet for life-threatening hemorrhage from an arm or a leg
  - Apply the tourniquet *above* the bleeding site, *over* the uniform, tighten until bleeding stops, and either move the casualty to cover or direct the patient to move to cover

- Airway management is generally deferred until the next phase of care (Tactical Field Care) because managing an obstructed airway takes time and exposes the responder to the threat or hazard

The number one medical priority in Care Under Fire is to stop life-threatening bleeding from an arm or a leg as soon as possible.

Early control of severe hemorrhage is critical because uncontrolled bleeding from a limb is the most frequent cause of *preventable* death.

Injury to a major blood vessel can quickly lead to shock and death. For example, a trauma patient who has sustained a complete femoral artery and vein disruption can bleed to death in as little as 3 minutes.

It is important to remember that in this phase of care (Care Under Fire), only *life-threatening* bleeding warrants intervention. Minor scrapes and lacerations that have minimal bleeding are addressed in the Tactical Field Care phase of care.

5.A. TRAUMA VICTIM INCIDENTS & HEMORRHAGE CONTROL

There are a number of steps to take whenever an incident occurs that involves one or more trauma victims.

First:

- Identify all of the injured victims
- Next identify the injured victims that are bleeding
- Finally, identify the injured victims that are bleeding a lot...those are the ones you want to deal with first

Next find the bleeding site:

- Sometimes it will be obvious.
- Victims with injuries to major blood vessels will often have blood spurting or flowing that is easily visible
- Sometimes you will have to search for the bleeding
    - Put on a pair of gloves and run your gloved hands over the patient in an orderly fashion, looking for blood on the gloves after each area of the body is checked
        - Run your gloved hands down the patient's arms and legs and then look at the gloves for blood
        - Run your gloved hands down the front of the chest and abdomen and then look at the gloves for blood
        - Run your gloved hands down the back of the chest and abdomen and then look at the gloves for blood
        - Run your gloved hands over the head and scalp and then look at the gloves for blood

Depending on the location of the wound and the phase of care that the situation allows, take the appropriate action to control ongoing bleeding

- If the bleeding is from a limb (arm or leg):
    - Control the bleeding by applying a recommended tourniquet
    - This intervention can be performed in Care Under Fire either by the victim themselves or by a partner
- If the bleeding is from one of the junctional locations (neck, axilla [armpit], groin):

- First apply direct pressure to the bleeding site using your hand or finger
    - Then pack the wound with a topical hemostatic gauze and apply pressure for the appropriate amount of time
    - Because this intervention takes time to perform and could expose the responder to the hazard or threat, it is performed during Tactical Field Care when the situation is safer

- If the bleeding is from a central location (chest, back, abdomen, flank):
    - Bleeding in these locations is typically internal and cannot be controlled in field
    - Identify these victims to arriving EMS personnel for rapid transport to trauma center
    - This is Tactical Evacuation care

5.B. LIMB (ARM, LEG) HEMORRHAGE

- Where a tourniquet can be applied, it is the *first* choice for control of life-threatening hemorrhage from an arm or leg
- Until the military experience in Iraq and Afghanistan, the use of tourniquets for bleeding from an arm or a leg was actively discouraged because of the concern for potential amputation of the limb due to the tourniquet
    - Review of data from Viet Nam and the Iraq/Afghanistan conflict revealed that the number one cause of preventable death was bleeding from an arm or a leg
    - As a result, the use of tourniquets was reconsidered.
    - The military undertook a major study of available tourniquets and developed criteria for what they wanted in a tourniquet:
        - The tourniquet had to be easy to apply one-handed in case one arm was injured and the other arm had to be used to apply it
        - The tourniquet had to be at least 1 ½ inches in width to minimize the potential for damage to underlying structures such as nerves and blood vessels
- The military then implemented training in tourniquet use
    - They found that 31 lives were saved in the first 6 months by the application of tourniquets

- It is estimated that over 2000 lives were saved with tourniquets in the first several years of use
- Most importantly, they found that ***No arms or legs were lost because of the application of a tourniquet***

As a direct result of the military experience, the following recommendations have been made:

- All public safety responders should carry a recommended tourniquet
- The tourniquet should be in a standard location on the uniform
- The tourniquet should be easy to access quickly
- Every public safety responder should be trained in tourniquet use

If a public safety responder becomes injured, he or she should be able to easily and quickly reach their *own* tourniquet.

Tourniquet Application – Key Points

- Apply the tourniquet to an arm or leg without delay for life-threatening external bleeding
- Apply the tourniquet, as high and as tight on the limb as possible, directly over the uniform
- Make sure the tourniquet is located above the bleeding site
- The tourniquet should be tightened until the bleeding is totally stopped
- The tourniquet should not be applied directly over:
  - joints (knee or elbow) – the bones of the joint will prevent it from compressing the blood vessels
  - a holster or other items on a duty belt
  - a pocket that contains bulky items
- Sometimes a second tourniquet may be needed to control bleeding, usually on a leg
  - The second tourniquet should be placed just above the first one
- If treating a buddy, use *their* tourniquet first and save your tourniquet for yourself unless they don't have one
- Training tourniquets should never be used as mission tourniquets
  - Repetitive training applications may cause tourniquet failure

Recommended Tourniquets

The U.S. Military has conducted extensive tests on the commercially available tourniquets and recommends the following tourniquets:

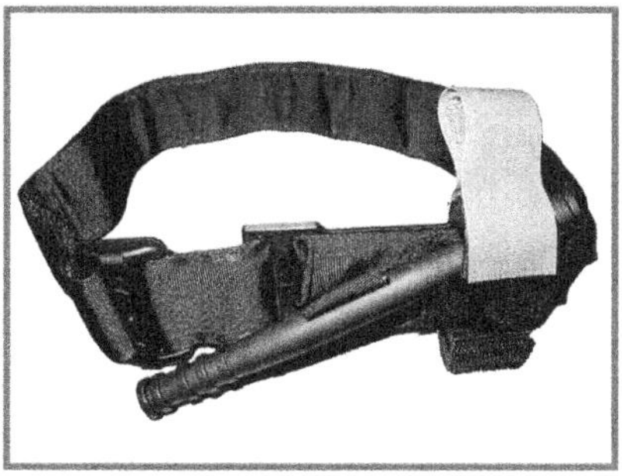

Combat Application Tq (CAT)

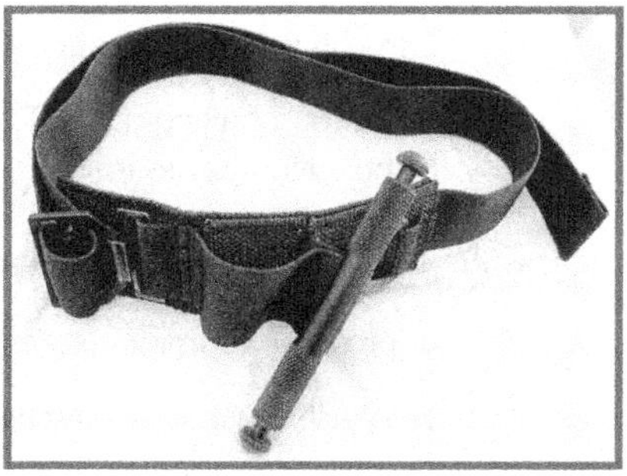

SOF Tactical Tq (SOFTT -Wide)

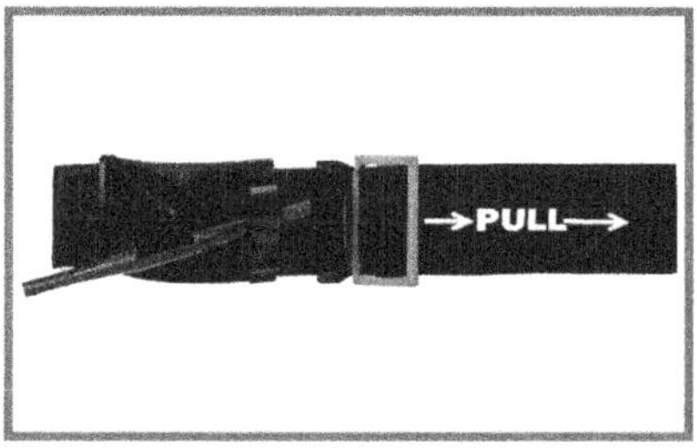

Tactical Mechanical Tq (TMT)

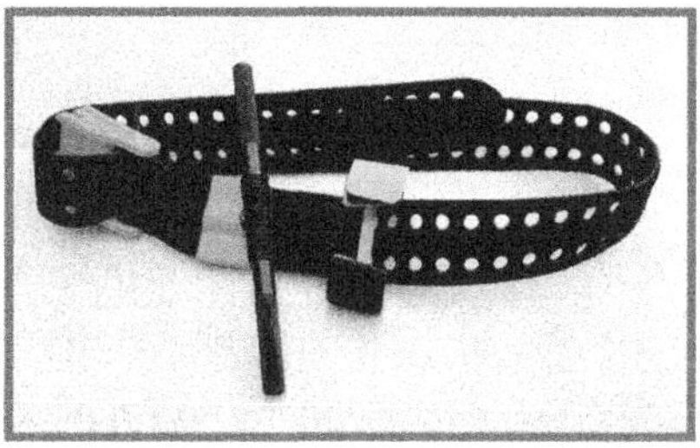

SAM XT Tq

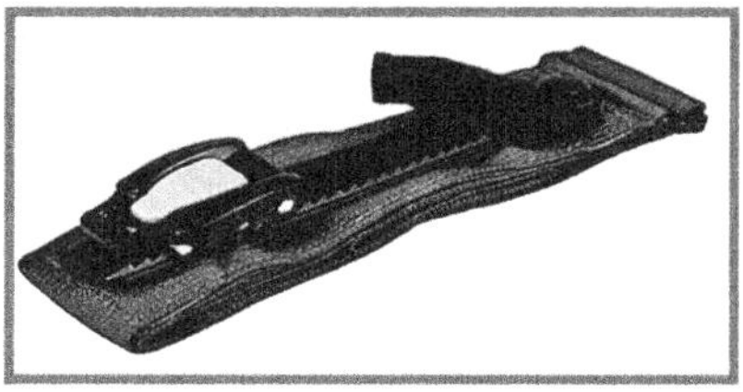

TX2 Tq

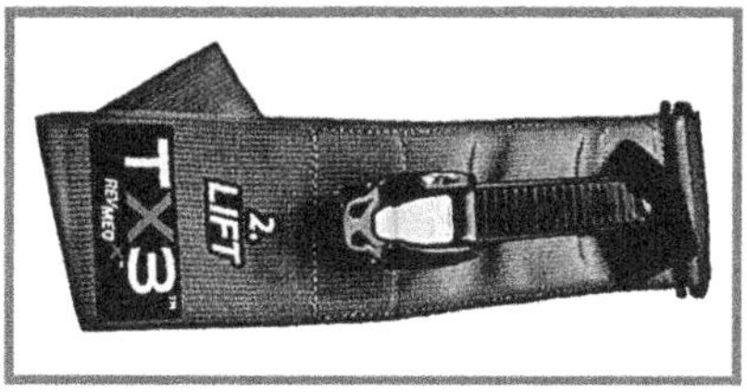

TX3 Tq

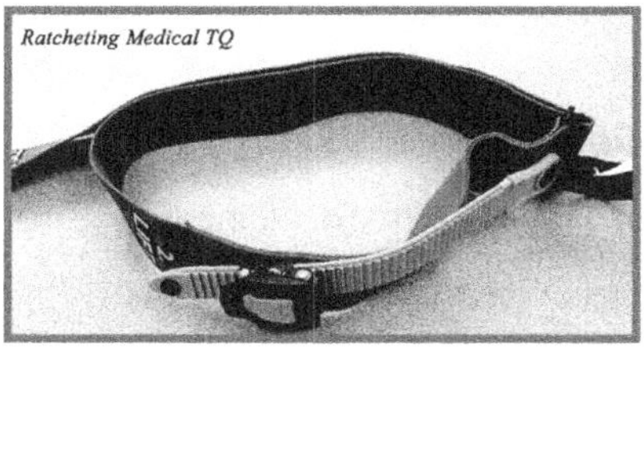

Order tourniquets from approved medical, law enforcement, or tactical equipment distributors.

- Counterfeit tourniquets are being manufactured and sold, especially the C.A.T.
    - The counterfeits are poor quality and prone to failure
    - When purchasing a C.A.T., ensure that you have this National Supply Number tourniquet: NSN 6515-01-521-7976
- What about improvised tourniquets?
    - Improvised tourniquets are generally *not* recommended
    - They are much less effective than commercially available tourniquets
    - They are difficult to make and effectively apply without extensive practice
    - Too much time is often spent trying to find the needed materials and to make one while the patient is bleeding
    - Most improvised tourniquets are too thin and narrow leading to damage of tissues underneath
    - A poorly made and applied improvised tourniquet will often increase the bleeding, rather than decrease it

Tourniquet Pain

- Tourniquets HURT when applied effectively…they hurt a lot
- Pain does not indicate a mistake in application
- Pain does not mean that the tourniquet should be removed
- When the situation allows, get EMS to the patient to manage pain with analgesics

Tourniquet Mistakes to Avoid

- Not using one when you should – the patient continues to bleed
- Using a tourniquet for minimal bleeding – while this is a mistake, if you are not sure if the bleeding is life-threatening, apply the tourniquet and then, as soon as possible, have EMS evaluate whether or not it was needed

- Putting the tourniquet on too high when you can see the wound – if the wound is easily visualized, the tourniquet may be placed 2-3 inches above the wound
- Removing the tourniquet when the casualty is in shock or has only a short transport time to the hospital – as a general rule, a tourniquet applied in the field should only be removed once the patient has been transported to the hospital/trauma center
- Not tightening the tourniquet enough to eliminate the distal pulse – when the situation allows, check to see that the pulse in the limb can no longer be felt. If a pulse is still felt, that means that blood is getting past the tourniquet, bleeding may still be occurring, and a limb-threatening condition called compartment syndrome may be developing. The tourniquet requires additional tightening or a second tourniquet should be applied.
- Not using a second tourniquet if needed – while one tourniquet will stop bleeding in most cases, occasionally, a second tourniquet may be needed. Typically, this will be on a leg. If a second one is needed, it should be applied next to and just above the first one
- Waiting too long to put the tourniquet on – this allows the victim to lose more blood and potentially develop shock
- Periodically loosening the tourniquet to allow blood flow to the injured extremity – for many years, it was taught that if a tourniquet was applied, the tourniquet should be loosened every 15 to 20 minutes to allow blood to flow back into the extremity and hopefully prolong the survival of the injured limb. Unfortunately, loosening the tourniquet permits additional blood loss which will lead to shock. Therefore, once tightened, a tourniquet should not be loosened

REMEMBER: Only life-threatening bleeding from an arm or a leg requires tourniquet application. Wound that are not bleeding *Do NOT* need a tourniquet.

Note the wounds in the two photos below – neither wound demonstrates life-threatening bleeding and therefore neither one requires tourniquet application.

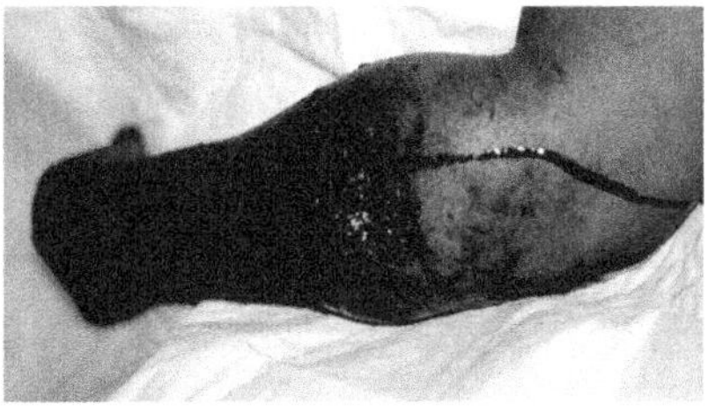

Shotgun wound with minimal bleeding

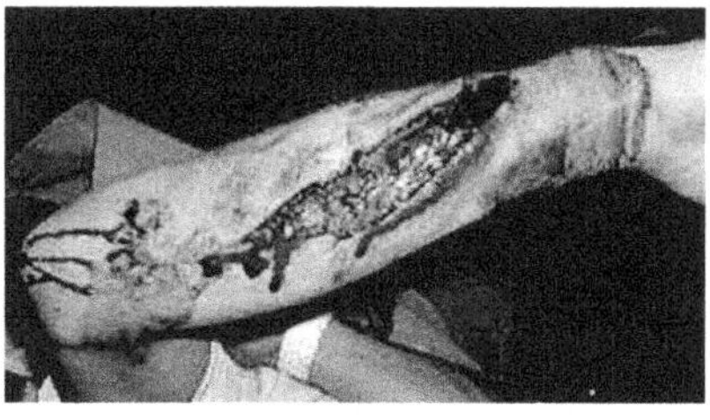

Forearm laceration with minimal bleeding

Tourniquet Application – the following series of steps demonstrate the application of the Combat Application Tourniquet (C.A.T.). If one of the other recommended tourniquets is used, the responder should be trained and practiced in the proper application of the selected device.

Step 1. Insert the wounded extremity (arm or leg) through the loop of the C-A-T

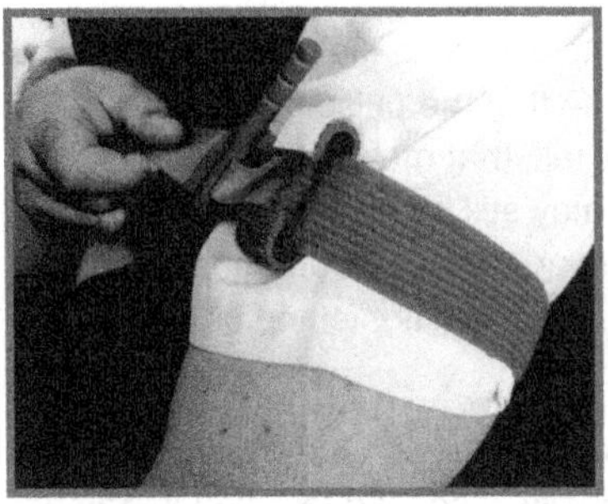

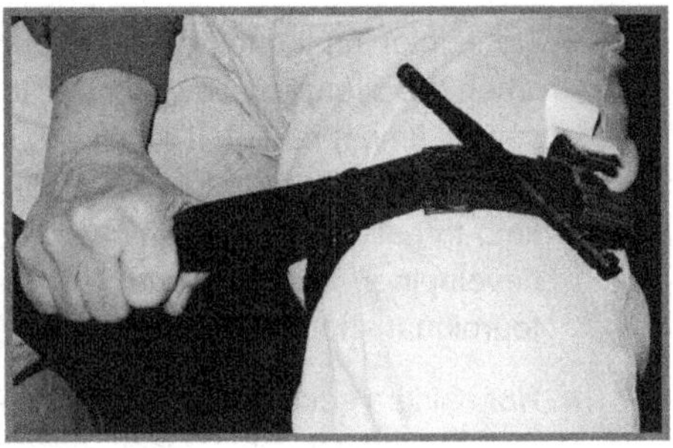

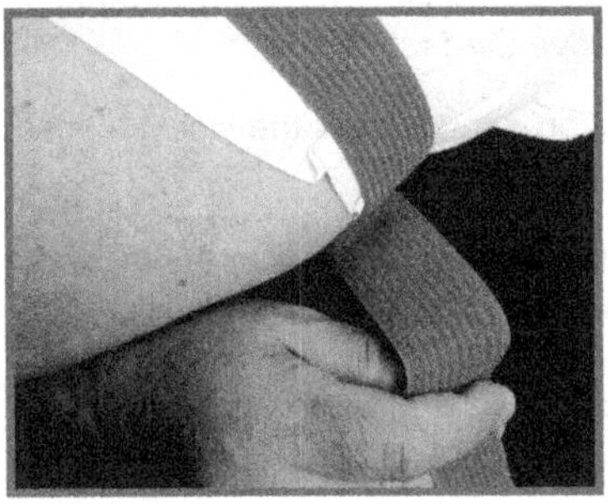

Step 2. Pull the self-adhering band as tight as you can, and securely fasten it back on itself. ***BE SURE TO REMOVE ALL SLACK FROM THE LOOP***

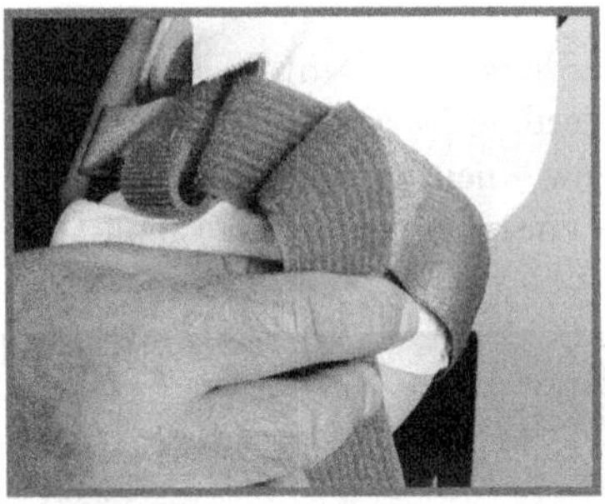

Step 3. Adhere the band around the extremity, just up to the clip.

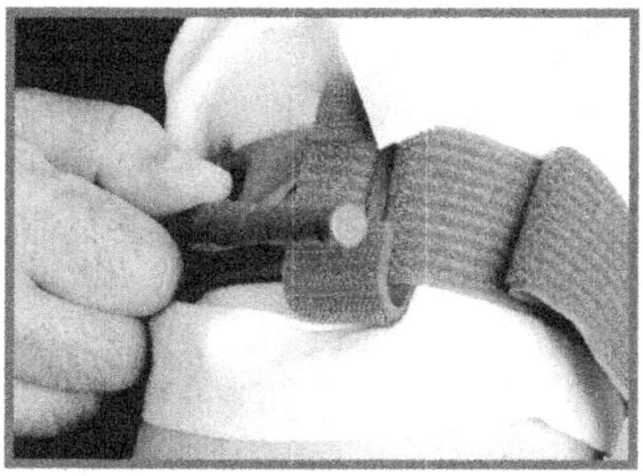

Step 4. Twist the windlass rod until the bleeding has stopped.

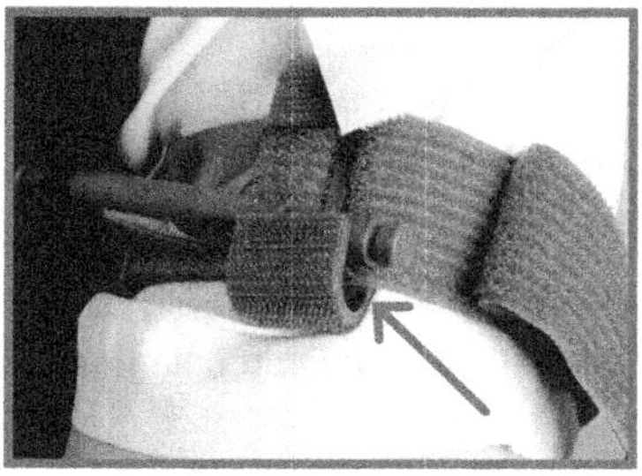

Step 5. Lock the windlass rod in place in the windlass clip. Bleeding is now controlled.

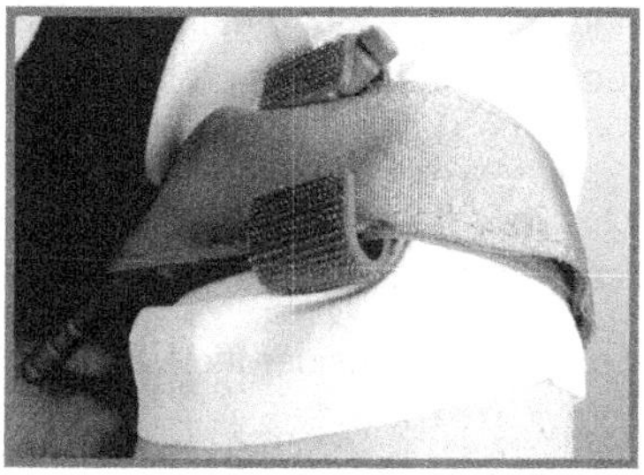

Step 6. Adhere the remaining self-adhering band over the rod, through the windlass clip, and continue around the extremity as far as it will go.

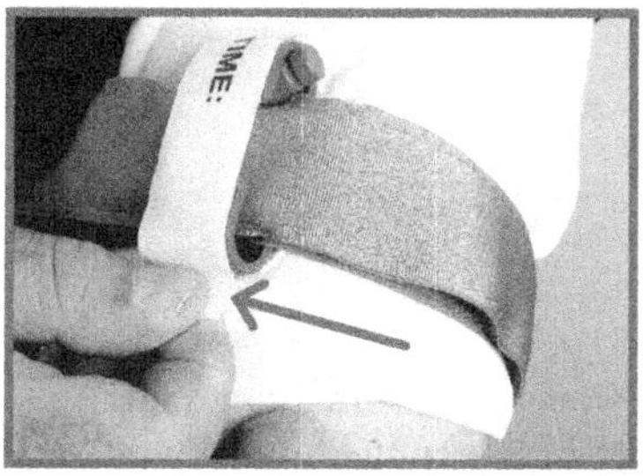

Step 7. Secure the rod and the band with the windlass strap. Grasp the windlass strap, pull it tight, and adhere it to the opposite hook on the windlass clip.

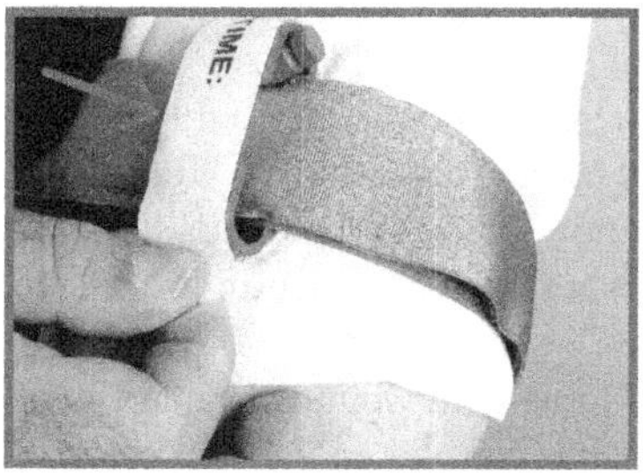

Step 8. Note the time the tourniquet was applied. If you have a marker, you can write it directly on the tourniquet. The patient is now ready for transport.

Care Under Fire involving an Active Shooter

- If the firefight is ongoing – don't try to treat the casualty in the *Kill Zone*! Treating a casualty in a "kill zone" is likely to lead to additional victims
- Suppression of hostile fire and moving casualties to cover are the major concerns
- Suppression of hostile fire will minimize the risk of both new casualties and additional injuries to the existing casualties

Care Under Fire - Moving Casualties to Cover

- If a casualty is awake and able to move themselves, he or she should move to cover on their own to avoid exposing rescuers to the threat
  - Often it may be necessary to direct or order a wounded individual to move since they may get focused on their injury and not on moving to a safe location
- If a casualty is not responsive or moving, it is likely that that individual is beyond help and attempting a rescue while under fire is probably not worth the risk
- If a casualty is responsive but unable to move for whatever reason, a rescue plan should be devised if tactically feasible
  - If you must move a casualty while under fire, consider the following:
    - Distance to be covered
    - Location of nearest cover
    - How best to move him to cover
    - The risk to the rescuers
    - Weight of casualty and rescuer

Care Under Fire and Junctional Wounds: Some wounds are located in places where a tourniquet cannot be applied. This particularly applies to the junctional locations: the neck, axilla (armpit), and groin. These injuries are usually treated by packing the wounds with a hemostatic agent (e.g., Combat Gauze™) or other dressing and applying direct pressure for the recommended amount of time. Treatment of junctional wounds generally is not tactically feasible in CUF because of need to hold direct pressure for at least 3 minutes, therefore potentially exposing the rescuer to the threat. Junctional wounds are treated in Tactical Field Care.

Care Under Fire and the Airway: Similar to junctional wounds, management of an obstructed airway takes time. As a result, it is considered too dangerous to attempt to manage it in Care Under Fire. Treatment of the airway is deferred until Tactical Field Care when the casualty has been moved to cover. If a casualty has no airway in the Care Under Fire phase, chances for survival are minimal. Importantly, death from compromised airways is relatively infrequent.

Care Under Fire and Spine Precautions: Someone familiar with standard EMS practice is aware that concern for vertebral spine and spinal cord injuries is something that is always at the forefront of the EMS responder's considerations for trauma victims. However there are a number of important changes in tactical situations:

- Penetrating Wounds (gunshots [GSW], stab wound [SW], shrapnel)
  - Penetrating injuries, regardless of cause, ***DO NOT*** require spine stabilization
  - In penetrating trauma, either:
    - the spinal cord is damaged at the moment of injury, or
    - The spinal cord was missed, in which case there is no risk of subsequent damage (unlike with blunt trauma, such as a motor vehicle crash)
    - In either case, spinal motion restriction is not required
- Blunt Trauma (falls, motor vehicle accidents)
  - Blunt trauma is different!
  - Neck or spine injuries due to blunt mechanisms of injury may require spinal motion restriction
  - Apply only if the danger of hostile fire does not constitute a greater threat

Care Under Fire - Summary of Key Points

- Control the threat and take appropriate cover!
- Direct or expect casualty to remain involved if able
- Direct casualty to move to cover if able
- Try to keep the casualty from sustaining additional wounds
- Stop life-threatening external hemorrhage if tactically feasible
  - Use a tourniquet for hemorrhage from an arm or leg
  - Direct casualty to control hemorrhage by self-aid if able
  - Junctional bleeding and airway management are generally deferred until the Tactical Field Care phase

6. TACTICAL FIELD CARE (TFC) - INDIRECT THREAT CARE

This section describes the recommended care to be provided in TFC. Tactical Field Care is distinguished from Care Under Fire by:

- A reduced level of hazard from a hostile or hazardous situation
- More time is available to provide medical care based on the tactical situation

Medical gear is still limited to that carried by the individual, medic or other responders. It may also include medical supplies and gear stored in tactical or other law enforcement vehicles.

The sequence of medical care priorities assumes that any obvious life-threatening arm or leg bleeding has been addressed in the Care Under Fire phase. If this is not the case – address any massive bleeding first.

Tactical Field Care may consist of rapid treatment of the most serious wounds with the expectation of a re-engagement with hazardous situation at any moment or there may be ample time to render whatever care is needed and possible in the field. Time to formal extrication and evacuation may vary from minutes to several hours or longer depending on securing the scene to allow such actions to take place.

As a reminder, the M.A.R.C.H. acronym defines the general approach to and priorities for prehospital medical care of a trauma patient.

- **M**assive hemorrhage

  Life-threatening bleeding should be controlled as soon as possible
- **A**irway

  An open airway should be established and maintained
- **R**espiration (Breathing)
  - Open chest wounds that are bubbling or sucking air should be sealed
  - A possible tension pneumothorax, which is a life-threatening problem, should be recognized and the suspicion reported immediately to arriving EMS responders
- **C**irculation

  All other bleeding should be controlled
- **H**ypothermia/**H**ead injury
  - Prevent/treat hypothermia (decreased body temperature)
  - Recognize the signs of a possible head injury

Key Point: Any armed casualty with an altered mental status, for whatever reason, should be disarmed immediately.

- Officers (or others) with an altered mental status after injury may use their weapons inappropriately
- Secure all weapons - long gun, handguns, knives
- Possible causes of altered mental status are traumatic brain injury (TBI), shock, and hypoxia (not enough oxygen getting to the organs of the body, especially the brain.)
- Explain to casualty: "Let me hold your weapon for you while you are examined"

6.A. TACTICAL FIELD CARE - AIRWAY MANAGEMENT - M.A.R.C.H.

Conscious casualty:
Allow the casualty to assume any position that they prefer and that best protects the airway, to include sitting up and leaning forward

Unconscious casualty:
The treatment of an unconscious trauma victim involves two steps:

1. Assess the airway
2. Open the airway if necessary

In order to assess the airway:

- ***Look*** for obvious trauma to the air passageways including the nose, mouth, and neck (trachea)
- ***Listen*** for noisy respirations including snoring, gurgling

  If noisy respirations are heard, this means that there is airway compromise or obstruction

Airway Obstruction

- The most common cause of airway compromise is the tongue. When the tongue is the case of airway obstruction, the result is snoring sounds
- Patients with altered mental status often cannot keep the airway open on their own, so the muscles of the tongue relax, the tongue falls back and blocks the airway

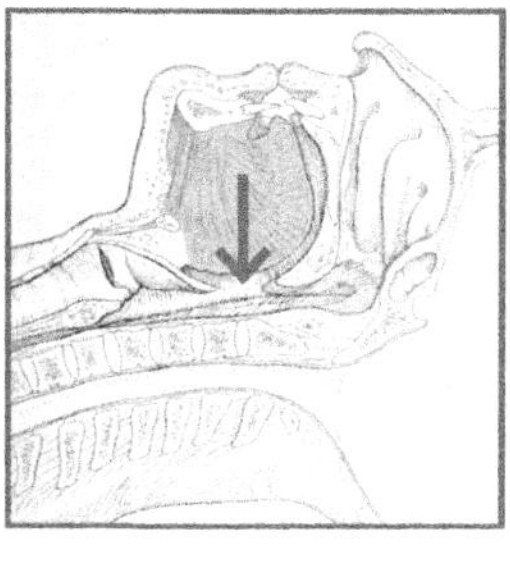

Opening the airway requires lifting the tongue from the back of the throat. The tongue is attached directly to the mandible (jawbone). Therefore, by lifting the mandible or jaw, the tongue can be lifted off the back of the throat and the airway opened. Successful lifting of the tongue is indicated when the snoring disappears.

Manual opening of the airway is accomplished by performing a procedure known as the Trauma Jaw Thrust.

Trauma Jaw Thrust

Step 1. Place your thumbs onto each of the patient's cheekbones.

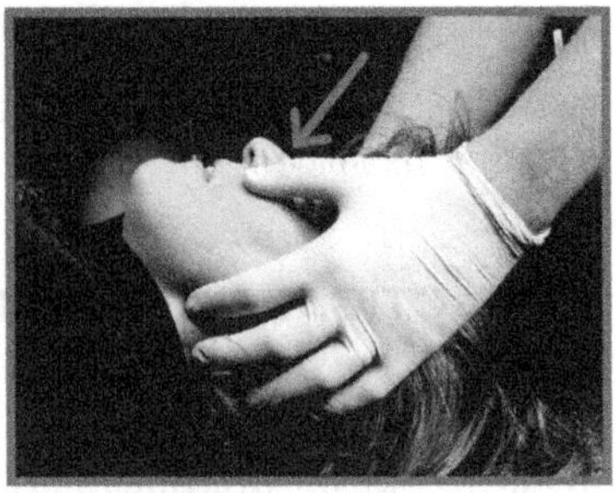

Step 2. Place your fingers along the bottom and back side of the mandible or jawbone.

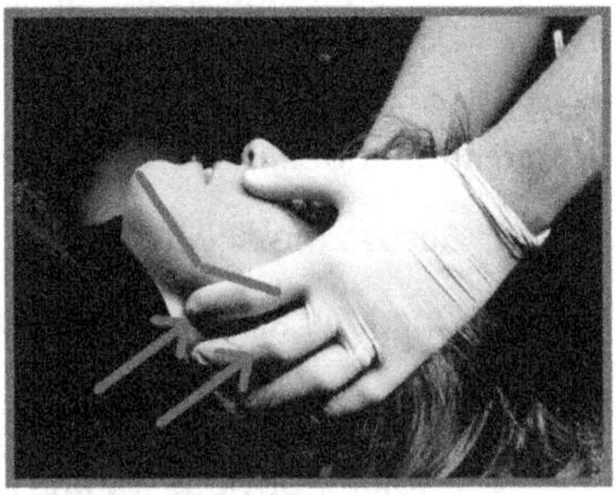

Step 3. Push the jawbone upwards toward the ceiling or sky. Listen for the cessation of snoring indicating that the tongue has been successfully lifted off the back of the throat and the airway has been opened.

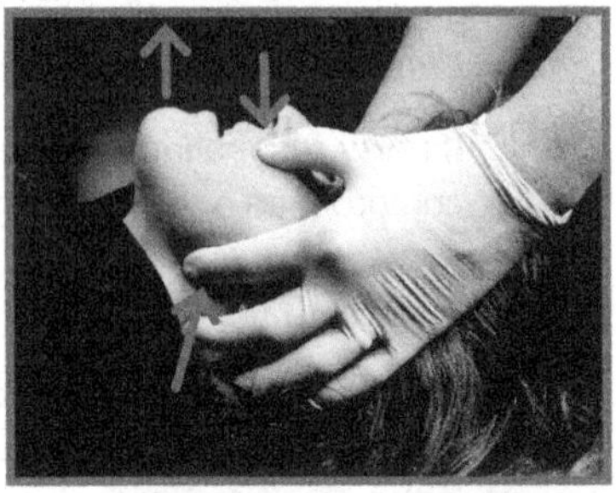

Step 4. After manually opening the airway, place unconscious casualties in the recovery position.

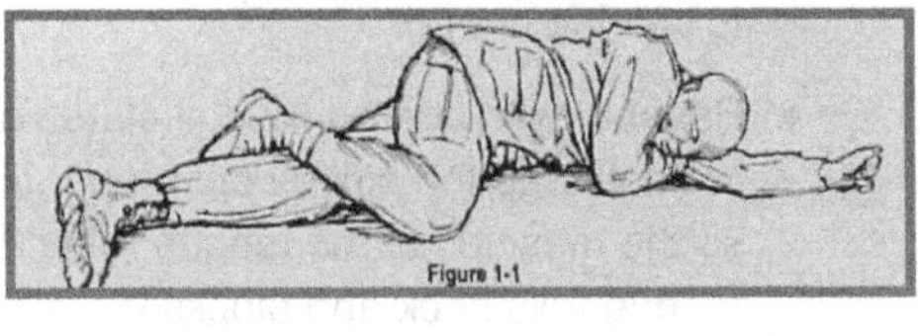

6.B. TACTICAL FIELD CARE - M.A.R.C.H. - RESPIRATIONS (BREATHING)

If an individual sustains either penetrating or blunt trauma involving the chest (front, back, or side), it is possible for the lung to be injured and cause difficulty breathing and shortness of breath. The lung on the damaged side can even collapse, either partially or completely. It is always important to assess how easily and well a trauma patient is breathing.

Pneumothorax

What does pneumothorax mean?

"Pneumo" = air
"Thorax" = chest

- Pneumothorax is air inside the chest cavity but outside of the lung

If you get shot, stabbed or get hit with a piece of shrapnel in the chest (front, back or side)...

- The penetrating object (bullet, knife, shrapnel) will go through your chest wall
- It will hit the lung underneath
- When it hits the lung, it will put a hole in the lung
- That hole will start to leak air outside of the lung but inside of the chest cavity - THAT is a pneumothorax

There are three types of pneumothorax:

- Simple
- Tension
- Open (sucking chest wound)

Simple Pneumothorax

- Most common type of pneumothorax
- Collection of air between the lung and chest wall causing the lung to collapse
- Usually not a big problem and does not require any specific treatment in the field

Tension Pneumothorax

- Tension pneumothorax is the second most common cause of preventable death after trauma in the military

- Tension pneumothorax may occur with wounds in chest as well as the upper abdomen, shoulder, or neck
- It may also occur as a result of blunt (i.e. motor vehicle accident) trauma but is less common
- In the case of a tension pneumothorax, the lung is leaking air (similar to a simple pneumothorax). But, in this case, the air leak continues and pressure begins to build up inside the damaged side of the chest. This causes the lung on that side to collapse completely and also causes the heart to shift towards the opposite side, thus impairing circulation. As the heart shifts, it begins to compress the other lung. As a result, both lung function and heart function are compromised causing respiratory distress and shock
- How will you recognize a tension pneumothorax?
    1. Patient with trauma to the chest, either:
        - Penetrating injury - stab wound, gunshot wound, shrapnel, or
        - Blunt trauma – i.e. car crash with fractured rib puncturing lung, and
    2. Increasing trouble breathing
    3. Respiratory rate increasing
    4. Increasing shortness of breath
    5. More and more trouble speaking
- Treatment is to relieve the pressure and let the trapped air escape
- Done by getting paramedic to patient (or the patient to the paramedic) to insert a needle into the chest

Sucking Chest Wound (Open Pneumothorax)

- Results from large open defects in the chest wall. If the hole is large enough, it may interfere with breathing because air will preferentially move in and out of the hole instead of in and out of the windpipe (trachea)

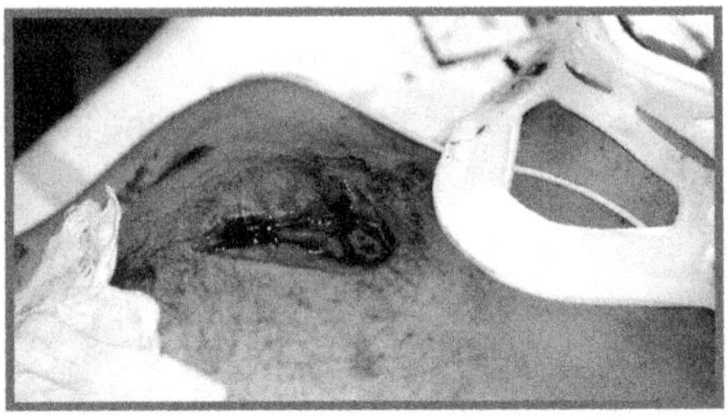

- Treat by applying an occlusive dressing, preferably a vented dressing, completely over the defect

- Allow the casualty to assume a position of comfort, including to be in the sitting position if breathing is more comfortable
- Monitor the patient for possible development of a subsequent tension pneumothorax
    - After treatment, a sucking chest wound can sometimes develop into a tension pneumothorax because the lung underneath is still leaking air and the chest has now been sealed with the dressing. This will allow pressure to build up within the chest.
    - When should this complication be considered?
    - When a patient with a sucking chest wound that has been treated starts to complain of more trouble breathing or is noted to have increasing respiratory difficulty.
- The treatment, as before, is to relieve the pressure but in this case a needle does not need to be inserted to allow the release of the air. Simply, pull off the covering bandage for 10-15 seconds, then reapply
    - aRemember - Tension pneumothorax is a common but easily treatable cause of preventable death. Recognize that it is happening and get paramedics to the victim (or the victim to the paramedic) as soon as possible!
    - How will you recognize it? Any patient who has sustained a penetrating wound of the chest *AND* has *increasing* trouble breathing

6.C. TACTICAL FIELD CARE - M.A.R.C.H. - CIRCULATION

- Assess the individual for any previously unrecognized hemorrhage and control all sources of external bleeding
- If not already done, use a recommended tourniquet to control life-threatening external hemorrhage from an arm or a leg or for any traumatic amputation
    - Apply the tourniquet directly on the skin 2-3 inches above wound
    - Reassess all previous tourniquet applications
    - Expose all wounds by removing or cutting open covering clothing
    - Look at the wound to determine if the tourniquet is still needed
    - If so, replace a tourniquet that was applied over the uniform or clothing with another one applied directly to skin 2-3 inches above wound

- If tourniquet is not needed, use other techniques such as direct pressure or wound packing to control bleeding
- Expose and clearly mark all tourniquet sites with the time of tourniquet application using an indelible marker

Tourniquet Points to Remember

- Damage to an arm or leg is rare if the tourniquet is applied for less than two hours
  - In fact, tourniquets are often left in place for several hours during surgery
- In the face of massive extremity hemorrhage, it is better to accept the small risk of damage to the limb than to have a casualty bleed to death
- When time and the tactical situation permit, check for presence or absence of a pulse beyond the tourniquet
- If a distal pulse is still present, the tourniquet is *NOT* tight enough
  - Consider additional tightening of the tourniquet or the use of a second tourniquet, next to and just above the first, to eliminate the distal pulse
  - Tightening the tourniquet enough to eliminate the pulse beyond the tourniquet will help to ensure that all bleeding is stopped
- Tightening the tourniquet enough to eliminate the pulse beyond the tourniquet will help prevent damage to the extremity from blood that enters the extremity but is not able to get out
  - What happens if blood can enter an extremity but not be able to get out?
    - Compartment Syndrome
      - The muscles in the arm and the leg are surrounded by a layer of thick, tough tissue that does not expand
      - This layer of tissue divides the limb into muscle compartments
      - If blood enters the compartment but cannot get out, the pressure inside the compartment will build up (much like a tension pneumothorax)
      - This will damage or cause the death of the muscle
      - This can be avoided by checking to see that the pulse is absent below the tourniquet

What do you do for bleeding from a site where you cannot place a tourniquet?

- For compressible hemorrhage in locations where a tourniquet cannot be applied, use a hemostatic agent to pack the wound and apply direct pressure
- If a hemostatic agent is unavailable, a standard gauze roll can be used very effectively
- After packing a wound, apply at least 3 minutes of direct pressure when using a hemostatic gauze or 10 minutes if using plain gauze

Junctional wounds are wounds that are located in the neck, axilla (armpit), or groin.

- A tourniquet cannot be applied to these locations
- In order to control bleeding from these sites, they need to be packed with a topical hemostatic gauze or plain gauze roll
- Once packed, direct pressure must be applied for the recommended amount of time
    - 3 minutes, minimum, if using a hemostatic gauze product
    - 10 minutes, minimum, if using a plain gauze roll
- This technique can control bleeding that might otherwise prove fatal

Hemostatic Gauze Agents – there are multiple products available:

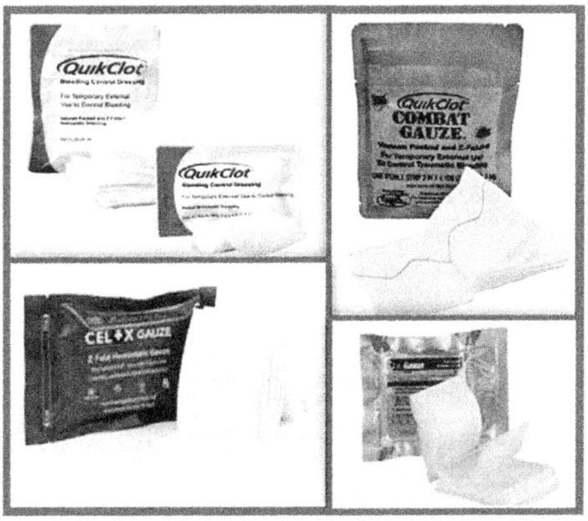

- Combat Gauze
- QuikClot
- Celox
- Celox Rapid
- Chitosan
- Chitogauze
- NuStat

All are products that are impregnated with an agent that promotes blood clotting and all are used in similar fashion.

At one time, there was a powder product that was poured into the wound. While it was effective in stopping bleeding, it produced a lot of heat when it reacted with blood...in fact, enough heat to cause significant burns to the patient. In the event you find a powder hemostatic product, ***DO NOT*** use it. These products are no longer recommended.

Wound Packing:

Step1. Open or remove clothing over the wound to expose the bleeding site.

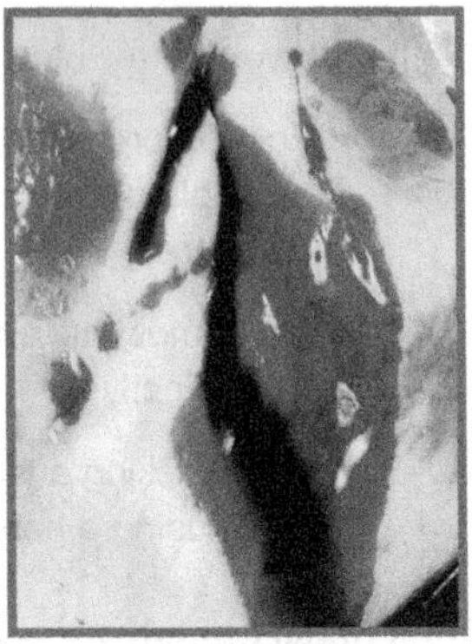

All wound packing images courtesy Rick Brady Photo

Step 2. If possible, gently remove or wipe away excess pooled blood from the wound while trying to preserve any clots already formed in the wound. Then, look in the wound and locate the source of the most active bleeding.

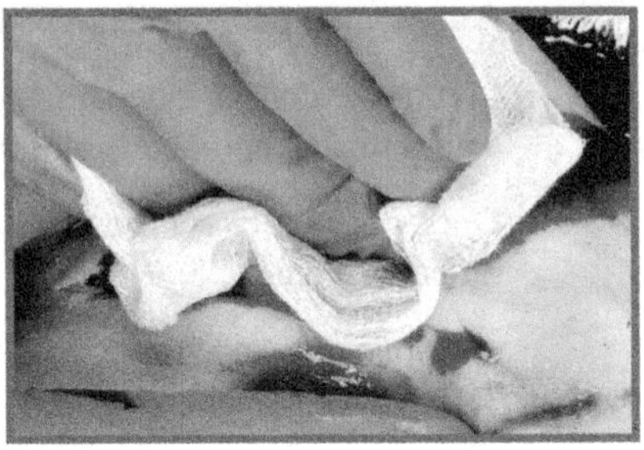

Step 3. Prepare to pack the wound, using:

- hemostatic dressing, OR
- plain gauze roll, OR
- a clean cloth if gauze is not available.

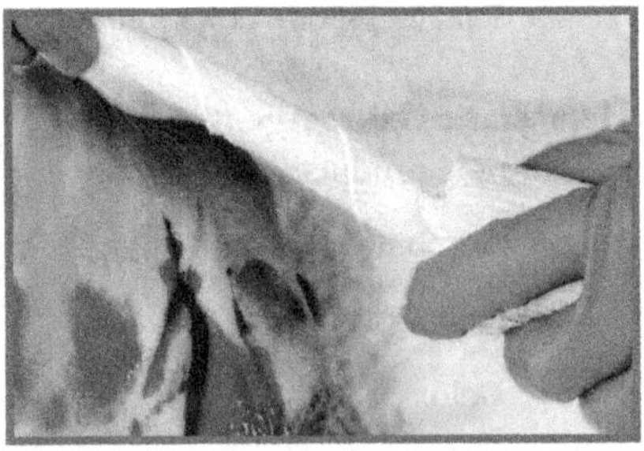

Step 4. Pack (stuff) the wound as deeply as possible, all the way down to the bottom, and directly onto the bleeding site.

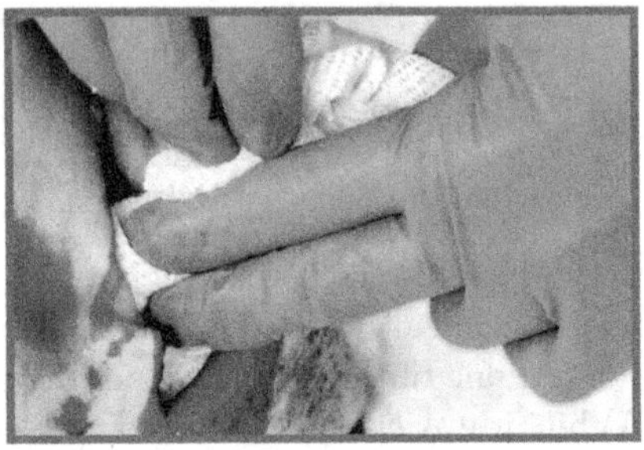

The upper two images demonstrate proper packing all the way to the bottom of the wound.

The lower two images show covering the wound but not packing it.

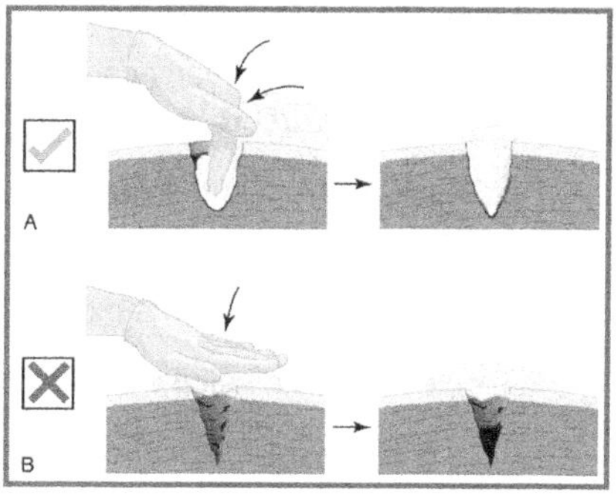

Step 5. Quickly apply and hold pressure directly on the packed wound until relieved by medical responders.

- Minimum 3 minutes for hemostatic gauze
- Minimum 10 minutes for plain gauze

Step 6. Secure the packing in place by wrapping with an elastic bandage or other wrap. Transport the patient and monitor for any resumption of bleeding.

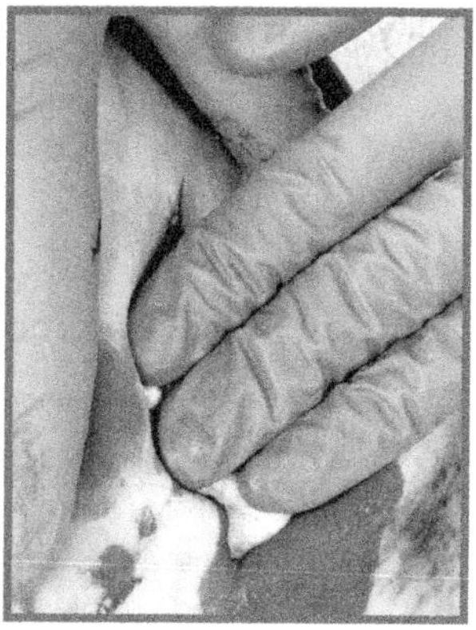

Direct Pressure

- The application of direct pressure on a bleeding wound can stop most hemorrhage, even if a hemostatic agent is not available
  - Direct pressure can stop even carotid and femoral bleeding
- Use your hand or fingers and push on the wound using your body weight
- Do not release pressure to check the wound until you are prepared to control bleeding with a hemostatic agent or a tourniquet

It is important to note that the patient cannot be moved while the application of direct pressure is being used.

6.D. TRAUMA AND SHOCK

- Shock can have many causes, but *in the trauma situation, it is* ***typically caused by severe blood loss***
- "Shock" is the result of inadequate blood flow to the body tissues. When this happens:
    - There is inadequate oxygen delivery to the cells of the body
    - As a result, cellular dysfunction occurs
    - Cellular dysfunction can lead to cell death
    - If enough cells die, the organ dies
    - If enough organs die, the patient will die
- This is why it is so important to stop on-going bleeding as soon as possible

How can shock be recognized in the field?

- Law enforcement and first responder personnel need a *fast, reliable, low-tech* way to recognize shock

    1. The brain is extremely sensitive to any decrease in oxygen or blood supply. As a result, the victim's mental state and level of consciousness will decrease and progress from normal to confusion and uncooperativeness to unconsciousness
    2. As more blood is lost, the body will try to compensate by increasing the heart rate to pump what blood is left to the organs

- Therefore, the best indicators of shock are:
    - Decreased state of consciousness (if casualty has not suffered head injury), and/or
    - Weak or absent radial pulse

CONTROL THE BLEEDING FIRST, before signs of shock appear, if at all possible

- Hemorrhage control takes precedence

Then, get the paramedic to the patient or the patient to the paramedic.

6.E. TACTICAL FIELD CARE - M.A.R.C.H. - HYPOTHERMIA

Prevent hypothermia - (decrease in body temperature)

- Try to minimize a casualty's exposure to the elements
- Keep protective gear on or with the casualty if feasible
- Replace wet clothing with dry if possible
- Get the casualty onto an insulated surface as soon as possible
- Use dry blankets, poncho liners, sleeping bags, or anything that will retain heat and keep the casualty dry

Key Point: Even a small decrease in body temperature can interfere with blood clotting and increase the risk of bleeding to death

- Casualties in shock are unable to generate body heat effectively
- Wet clothes increase body heat loss
- Remove wet clothes and cover casualty dry clothing or blankets

Key Point: Hypothermia is much easier to prevent than it is to treat!

6.F. TACTICAL FIELD CARE - PENETRATING EYE TRAUMA

- If the eye is struck by a piece of shrapnel or other foreign body, a penetrating eye injury must be suspected
- **DO NOT RUB OR PUT ANY PRESSURE ON THE EYE**
    - If any of the contents of the eye are extruded, they cannot be replaced. The eye will lose its round shape and vision will be permanently impaired or lost

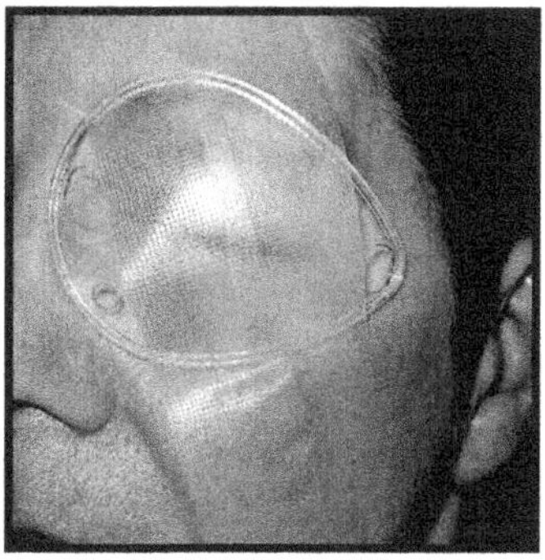

- Perform a rapid field test of visual acuity
- Determine if the casualty:
    - Can read print
    - Count fingers
    - See hand motion
    - Has light perception
- Cover the eye with a rigid eye shield (NOT a pressure patch)

6.G. TACTICAL FIELD CARE - CARDIOPULMONARY RESUSCITATION (CPR)

- Victims of blast or penetrating trauma who have no pulse, are not breathing, and no other signs of life are dead
    - Resuscitation will not be successful and should not be attempted
- When should you consider performing CPR?
    - When the cause of cardiac arrest is from something OTHER THAN trauma, such as:
        - Heart attacks
        - Hypothermia
        - Electrocution
        - Other non-traumatic causes
- Why shouldn't CPR be performed?
    - Doing CPR exposes the responder to the threat or hazard
    - CPR performers may get killed
    - The primary mission gets delayed
    - The casualty stays dead

Tactical Field Care - Further Elements

- Reassess the victim regularly for any recurrence of bleeding, trouble breathing, etc.
- Prepare the victim for transport
- When EMS arrives...
    - Tell them:
        - what injuries you saw,
        - what you did to manage those injuries, and
        - any changes in the casualty's status

Tactical Field Care - Summary of Key Points:

Care is still being provided in a potentially hazardous environment

- Medical resources are still limited to what you carry on your person

- Hemorrhage control remains the priority
- Obstructed airways should be opened
- Breathing problems should be identified
    - Sucking chest wounds (open pneumothorax) should be sealed
    - Tension pneumothorax should be recognized and immediately referred to a paramedic
- Prevent hypothermia
- Place a rigid eye shield for any suspicion of a penetrating eye injury
- No CPR for victims of trauma
- Provide a verbal report of your findings and care to EMS

7. TACTICAL EVACUATION CARE - EVACUATION CARE

- The threat or hazardous situation has been completely controlled or contained.
- The appropriate medical interventions have been performed in Care Under Fire and Tactical Field Care
    - If not, they are accomplished now
- The patient is transferred to EMS for further treatment and transport to the appropriate destination

8. SUMMARY

Remember:

- The TCC-LEFR guidelines are not a rigid protocol that is written in stone
- The tactical or hazardous environment may require some modifications to the guidelines
- Think on your feet!

Goals for TCC for LEFR

- Stabilize the hazardous situation so EMS can come in and treat the patient

If that is not possible:

- Evacuate the patient to a location where they can safely receive care by EMS

If that is not possible:

- Provide treatment for life-threatening medical problems
    - Stop the bleeding
        - Tourniquet
        - Wound packing and pressure
    - Open an obstructed airway
    - Recognize increasing trouble breathing

Care Under Fire:

- Control the threat
- Move the casualty to cover
- Stop life-threatening bleeding from an arm or a leg
- Tourniquet
    - Self-aid or buddy aid

Tactical Field Care:

- Be sure life-threatening bleeding is controlled

    - Control bleeding of wounds that cannot have a tourniquet placed
    - Wound Packing and application of direct pressure
- Open an obstructed airway
    - Jaw Thrust
- Recognize worsening difficulty breathing
    - Need to get EMS in to treat tension pneumothorax

Tactical Evacuation Care:

- Tactical threats are controlled
- Casualty can be turned over to EMS
- Standard EMS treatment and transport

9. INDIVIDUAL FIRST AID KIT (IFAK)

- Strong consideration should be given to obtaining an IFAK for every responder

Examples of IFAKs

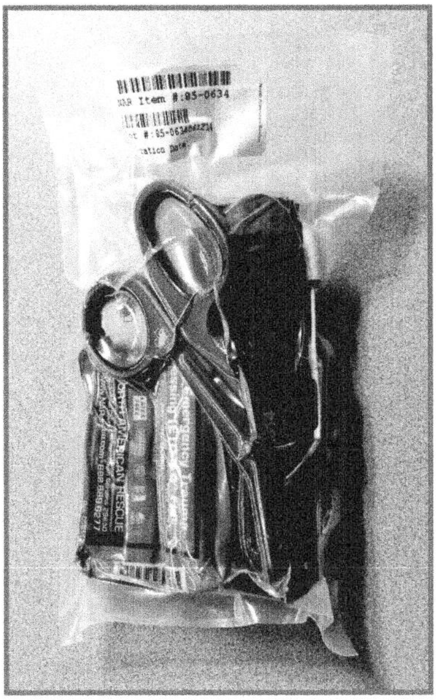

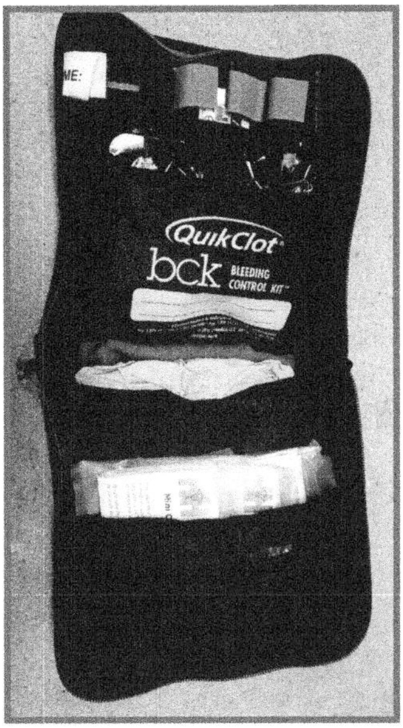

Typical IFAK Contents

- C.A.T. Tourniquet
- Gloves
- Shears
- Gauze roll
    - Plain or hemostatic
- Trauma bandage

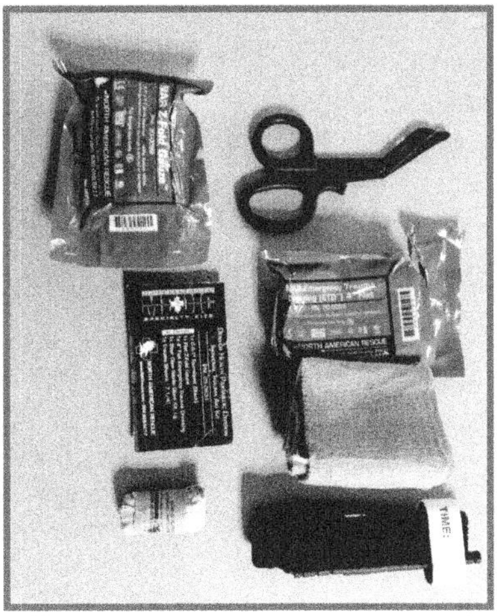

Civil disturbances are an all too common occurrence. These events may become violent resulting in traditional traumatic injuries to responders, participants, and innocent bystanders. These incidents may also cause injuries from other, less common causes including lasers, fireworks, and exposure to gas, smoke, and sometimes bodily fluids and substances. The Casualty Care for Civil Disturbances (CCC-D) educational program describes these various injuries and reviews their management. This course is appropriate for all public safety responders, especially law enforcement, who may be asked to respond to, and intervene at, civil disturbances.

Available as a half day educational course through the International Prehospital Medicine Institute. Accompanying monograph is available as an ebook or in paperback.

Made in the USA
Monee, IL
04 November 2026

67384265R00036